How To Powerlift

Learn To Squat, Bench, And Deadlift

By Polymath Power

Copyright

Table of Contents

The Problem

For many people, getting into training is hard. There are no two ways around this. You might be someone who has never set foot in a gym before. You may even be someone who has never considered how their current lifestyle can affect vital things such as posture, metabolism and eating habits.

This lifestyle can result in low energy, little patience, and little motivation to then finish a 9-5 shift and drive across town on a rush hour and hit a gym for a difficult and draining session.

For the people who are in this situation, they may find themselves in a position where they have the 9-5 job, followed by a school run, then a family meal so that they simply can not make the time to get themselves to the gym. The people with lifestyles such as this who do manage to make it to a gym are then most in need of finding a way to make every minute count.

Without knowing how to best use your time, you may find yourself unsure of what to do. You want to get stronger and fitter, but you end up spending the majority of the time on cardio machines or doing exercises for muscles in isolation, rather than compound movements which could help your overall issues such as posture and strength. You manage to stick with this routine for a year and enjoy the 'escape' offered by the gym from everyday life is pleasant but you still don't see the changes you want, you're still lateral raising the same weights as 8 months previously. As a result, you find yourself losing motivation to go even more so.

You may be the type of person who wants to get stronger but only knows how to train for looks. You may result in looking better but not actually feeling or being stronger. This is normally fine, but if we go back to the example of the office worker who needs posture and lifestyle improvements, you may need to add in some more specific strength work.

Focusing on the wrong things in the gym, or not making it to the gym at all can result in simple, everyday tasks becoming difficult. Try to pick something up off of the floor and then assess how you did it. Did you pick it up like you were taught to in your health and safety seminars in work? Or did you just bend down haphazardly with your heels raised and next to no balance involved? If it was more like the latter then you may need to focus on the proper movements (the squat, the deadlift, etc). You may think this doesn't affect your everyday life, but imagine picking your child up off of the floor, getting yourself off the couch or toilet, or even, carrying your shopping home. Better movements and strength will help with these everyday tasks.

Now that you've agreed that you can use a plan to get you stronger you decide to aim for your favorite strength athlete and follow their routine. You try it, you get a little stronger at first, but then you find yourself fatigued and not enjoying it. You may even find yourself struggling to fit it all in. The fact is, if you're a beginner you do not need fancy movements or workouts that push the gym's opening times to the limits. What you need is to focus on the basics, and get incredibly good at them. How you get good at them is highly individual and this is why copying someone who has already long gone through this process isn't viable.

A good routine is one in which you can set goals for the future and see yourself moving towards them. Again, this needs to be suited to you, Eddie Hall's deadlift plan to pull 500kg will be massively different from yours focusing on getting your first 1.5x bodyweight deadlift. Training towards your own specific goals and at your own specific time frame will result in your developing mentally also. However, a bad training plan could result in you becoming demotivated and see you leaving it all behind.

The Solution

Powerlifting. That is what this book is about, and it's probably what you want to get into (if you've read this far). Powerlifting focuses upon the increase of strength in the body but also in the mind, a good program is hard and requires a level of mental fortitude and determination that may be hard to come by in other aspects of life.

A good powerlifting program could be as infrequent as 3 days a week and still see you making gains. The reason for this is that it's so focused upon basic movements that you can get your sessions done within an hour in most cases.
Due to the massive compound movements involved you will hit pretty much every muscle group in one go, meaning that the amount of muscle you can affect in a short space of time is also increased greatly.

The simplicity of each movement also means that anyone can do it, regardless of age, gender or skill level. This also comes into effect in competitions, it doesn't matter if you're lifting 25kg or 250kg, you will receive the same level of support.

In the Problem section, we spoke about how most people will need more than just isolation exercises and cardio to improve their posture. The muscles involved in the big 3 power lifts are vital to posture, so if you get stronger at powerlifting you are likely to:

- Improve your posture
- Get stronger
- Move better
- Feel better
- Build more muscle
- Lose fat
- Develop a better habit driven lifestyle
- Focus better
- Increase confidence

Want to know how to achieve all of these? Simply read on.

Who Will Benefit From This Book?

This book has been written with a number of people, or groups, in mind. These people range from...

The complete beginner - Whether that be a beginner in terms of the gym or a trainer who has focused on aesthetics or cardio.

The trainer with no time - If you are struggling for time you want something that you *know* is going to help you. This book can guide you.

Those of you who want to build size, strength and muscle and bone density - Powerlifting will do exactly that, and this book will show you to do powerlifting.

Athletes who want to increase their performance -There are very few sports in the world where being stronger is a weakness. You are likely to excel further at your sport with added strength.

Advanced powerlifters or people who coach them - This book can act as a refresher course to those weathered by the experience of powerlifting.

Introduction to Powerlifting

Powerlifting is the pursuit of strength in the 'Big 3', which is, the squat; the bench press, and; the deadlift. These are three of the biggest compound lifts that you can do. This means that they employ more than one muscle group in order to work. By focusing upon these three lifts (with some accessory work thrown in) you will make your body exceptionally strong.

The Squat: To put it simply the squat is where you place a barbell across your upper back and then lower your hips to a point where your hip is below the top of your thigh(/knee, depending on the federation you compete in). This exercise relies upon great thigh and back strength.

The Bench Press: The king of the gym lifts. The bench is a very good upper body strength and size developer for anyone. It is where you lie down on a bench, unrack a barbell and then lower it to your chest and then lift it back to its starting position, then you re-rack it under the judge's command.

The Deadlift: Anyone who has been to a powerlifting competition will tell you that the competition doesn't truly start until the deadlifts have begun. The reason for this is that it is often the biggest lift of the big 3. The weight that this adds to your total can be huge.
A deadlift is basically where you pick up a barbell off of the floor and raise it until your knees, hips, and shoulders are locked out.

The Importance Of These Lifts

Powerlifting is all about getting as big a total across the three lifts as possible. However, training for these three lifts will result in big benefits in other areas of your life.

The squat will improve your leg strength, mobility, and even your posture. A strong butt and pair of legs are fantastic for standing up straight.

The bench press will help you develop a chest and a set of upper arms/shoulders that can make wearing a short-sleeved topless of a nightmare for you.

The deadlift basically teaches you how to safely pick things up off of the floor. Bending down to retrieve something is one of the most common ways to injure yourself, learn to do it right and get strong at it and you'll protect yourself from injury for years to come.

Gym Archetypes

A quick search online and you will see just how much of a line there is between each camp of lifter, whether that be a powerlifter, a crossfitter, a bodybuilder or an Olympic lifter. It's all a bit bizarre when you consider that they're all doing very similar things. However, despite their similarities, it is often easy to distinguish between the styles with a little information.

Powerlifters – This group will have a focus more on overall strength (with a side focus on shortening range of motion) when they are training. They can often be spotted with a different pair of shoes for squats, bench press, and deadlift, as well as a heavy-duty weight lifting belt, knee sleeves/wraps and a pair of wrist wraps.

Bodybuilders – These guys will keep a focus more on muscle growth, with a bit of a focus on strength gain too. They are likely to spend more time on smaller muscle groups than their powerlifting cousins, in order to achieve the most aesthetically pleasing, and most massive, muscle gain they can.

Olympic Lifters – These guys will look big and strong but might not do the traditional exercises you'd expect to see in a gym. They will be hoisting great big weights overhead, squatting deep and then dropping the weights from a height. They're meant to do this, it's not obnoxious, it's safe.

Crossfitters – Not to be confused with the Olympic lifters. They will use some of the Olympic style exercises but then they will use them in more a cardio or complex style of training.

Out of all of these groups, the powerlifters are likely to have a more focused routine in the gym, especially for beginners. At an early stage in training, you are likely to be focusing upon the technique of the big 3 lifts. You might only be training one to three different exercises per workout but you'll do so in such a way that you will improve on technique and strength in an optimal, time efficient manner.

The Benefits of Powerlifting

Strength and Confidence

The most obvious benefit of powerlifting would be the improvement of your physical strength. With this will also come more muscle and, if your diet allows, less fat. So you will not only be stronger, but you'll look it too.

This feeling of progress will then lead to a significant gain in your mental strength too. Your confidence will go up, you'll feel like a badass after smashing out a bench personal best that you couldn't even think of three months prior. This feeling of badassery will also reflect outwardly – you'll look like a badass too.

Functionality

There seems to be a commonly held belief that any kind of strength training will lead to being a musclebound oaf with no mobility, sense of space or depth and a complete lack of balance. However, this just is not true, in fact, it is quite the opposite which is true.

The mobility required to properly have a lift passed in this sport is of a very high standard. The muscle control and strength required will mean that your balance could improve also (or at least it'll hurt less if you fall over). The spatial awareness may just be on you though...

Health

Obviously, getting stronger means more muscle, probably less fat and a greater feeling mentally. But one thing that often gets ignored is the results in terms of bone health also.

Any high impact training will result in an increase of bone density. This can be massively important for as we grow older, particularly for ladies as they are more susceptible to osteoporosis and osteopenia (which is basically where the bone loses density and becomes brittle). Even if you were to show signs of osteoporosis in later life, the increased bone density you would have built up would mean that you're already ahead of it.

Another benefit, in a similar vein to bone density, would be the effect it can have on joint health. Strengthening the body through certain motions can lead to better control and if you have any issues like hypermobility in certain joints, learning how to properly move and strengthen and stretch in the correct areas could lead to you improving your health in that manner. Hypermobility can lead to a lot of pain and discomfort, especially if it goes to the extreme and leads to bone breaks or dislocations, so fixing or limiting this can be a massive health benefit.

Community

One of the biggest draws of powerlifting is the community behind it. Sure, training alone and getting big, strong and scary looks really cool but when you get to a competition you're surrounded by some of the most supportive people you will ever meet. This also goes for powerlifting clubs and teams, they act as a support network for you throughout your training, through the good times and the bad. A good team of lifters can be the most inspiring element you can add to your training.

You will definitely hear of stories of lifters going to pull a third attempt on deadlift while the person they're about to beat is watching on. In all of these stories in powerlifting the person at the side will be cheering as loud and as hard as anyone else in that room. That is the level of support you should expect in powerlifting.

The competition itself is comprised of three different exercises and three attempts at each lift. The competitions go by what is known as a 'raising bar,' this means that the lowest weight goes first and rises from there. This is applicable for the individual lifter, in that each attempt has to be higher than the last, and for the competition as a whole, as the attempts go in order of lowest to highest weight. Your highest achieved attempt in each lift is then added towards your total and the highest total wins.

The caveat to this is in Wilks based competitions. Wilks is basically a strength: bodyweight score. If two lifters score a 700kg total but one weighs 99kg and the other weighs 103kg, the 99kg has the higher Wilks score and is stronger.

The Mindset of Powerlifting

Powerlifting isn't just about getting bigger and stronger on a physical basis. It is analogous to many problems and issues in life, in that it can teach you how to use hard work, smart preparation and the support of others in order to achieve your goals.

In powerlifting, and in life, you need to be able to know when you should just keep plugging away at something or when you should strip it all back and really focus upon the basics of it all.

Do you need to focus on out and out strength? Or do you need to lower the weight and really teach yourself the movement pattern?

These questions come up in many areas of life, sometimes you can't answer them yourself but you need someone else there to monitor it and help you with how to proceed.

Powerlifting also requires mental toughness. Not only is it hard to get stronger in terms of what to do, but actually just doing it can be tough. You might be looking at going into the gym to squat for the 4th time this week, you know you can physically do it, but you need to get your head into mentally. You might be reading this thinking "I love squatting, that's fine," but imagine you're at the end of an intensity cycle before a big competition and everything just *hurts*. You need to be able to push on and carry on with your training.

This toughness, this perseverance is possibly the most important lesson you'll learn from powerlifting, and it can filter into your everyday life too.

You need to be able to come at training, and competing, from a wholesome position. If you've only focused upon one or two of the lifts in training then one of your lifts and your overall total are likely to suffer. If you haven't focused on your mindset going into this competition phase then you are going to find it hard to do any of it. Each competition, scratch that, each training session is an opportunity to learn something new about yourself in terms of the best way to compete, or the best way to be when lifting. How you manage yourself mentally is massively important. You might find you're the type to get aggressive and worked up before a lift, you might find you're chilled and laid back. Whatever works for you is highly individual and I'd strongly encourage you to play around with it and see. Copying your favorite lifter is all well and good but if it's not optimal for you, you're leaving KGs on the platform.

Learning about yourself like this, while also improving yourself, needs to be done on a completely consistent basis. If you do not give yourself the time or the focus required to get in the gym, put in the work and evaluate then you are selling yourself short.

It doesn't matter how naturally strong you are or how big your potential is, you need to be consistent. Work on your strengths, work on your weaknesses and do it week in, week out.

You will find that many places have started opening up powerlifting teams or clubs. These are usually run by a coach, preferably one with plenty of platform experience, and have a wide mixture of novice-intermediate-elite lifters within their ranks. A coach will be a massive help to a lifter of any level, they remove the worry of what to do while also providing the cues and encouragement to go on and perform to the best of your ability. The support of the fellow members is very, very important also. Whether you are lifting 25kg or 250kg, your team members will be there to support you through it, they're likely to be at the platform side cheering you on, whether you're about to take their records or not.

The "Big 3" Lifts

The Squat

The squat is an exercise that requires mobility, flexibility, strength, and control. As with all the lifts in Powerlifting, it is very individual:- it can be varied with bar position or foot width.

Bar Positions: There are two distinct bar positions which can be used with a squat:

1. High bar
2. Low bar

High Bar: The majority of people will learn high bar, and this will be in the inventory of the recreational gym goer too. High bar is where the bar is placed across the trapezius muscle near the neck. This position works best for people who squat with their back in a more upright position.

Low Bar: Low bar can be a bit more tricky to find the best position. The best way to find the correct position is to set the bar up in a high bar position against the rack and to slide the bar down your back until you find a second racking position, you'll feel where it sits nicely. With the bar being in this position you may find that your hand width is effected. You will likely also notice that your wrists, elbows, and shoulders will feel a little uncomfortable due to the rotation needed to grasp the bar correctly.

Genetics play a large role in which bar position you choose.

- High Bar requires – greater ankle flexion, shorter relative femur length, longer torso length, wider stance, and more quadriceps dominance.
- Low Bar requires - longer relative femur length, shorter torso, narrower stance, greater gluteal strength.

Footwear

High bar squats respond best to an elevation in the heel, so this is where weightlifting shoes can come in handy. Low bars respond better to no heel elevation, so flat shoes are good for this.

The Bench Press

The powerlifting bench press may look different compared to what you see most people do at the gym.

In a gym, you may see people doing bench with their feet up on the cushion, without the bar touching their chest or with a minuscule pause, if any. On a platform what you will see is a controlled descent of the bar down to the chest, sometimes on an arched back, followed by a press starting with a push from the legs in which the bar follows a particular bar path.

The Arch: The reasons for this is that in powerlifting you are trying to move the most weight over as short a distance as possible. You need to wait for a start command (when your arms are locked out with the bar held), a press command (after the bar has steadied upon your chest) and then a rack command (when the bar has returned to the start position).

Having an arch here means that the time between the start and the press command can be shortened as the bar only has to travel a matter of inches. Your hand width also plays a large role here.

Hand Position and Bar Path: You tend to see many lifters going for a close grip at first. This is because they are relying upon their arms, namely their triceps, in order to shift the bar to the right place. This can work but it also largely ignores the largest muscles involved – the pectorals.

The mechanics of the bench press mean that when the bar initially 'breaks' off of the chest, it is the chest muscles doing so, after this point it is then the shoulders which help out, and then finally the triceps locking the arms out with the bar over your face.

In order to fully take advantage of this 'roadmap' of muscles to be used, you should focus upon your bar path. The bar should come off of your chest and go up and then back and up, in an almost 'reverse J' shape. If you get this bar path correct you are taking advantage of your muscles proper biomechanics and should, therefore, be stronger with some work.

The Deadlift

The deadlift is quite often the powerlifter's largest lift. It is what really adds to their total. So much so that many people refer to the deadlift being where the competition really starts.
 As well as this being due to the sheer weight of most deadlifts, it is also due to the rules. Under IPF rules you can change your last deadlift attempt as many times as you like up to a minute before you lift, this may not sound like much but it can mean that you entice another lifter to try more than they can lift, resulting in them failing, only for you to lower your attempt and complete it. This makes it the most tactical point of the competition.

For you to do a deadlift, all you'll need is a barbell and plates, flat shoes (or socks/slippers) and maybe a belt and maybe some chalk. You can use straps, but most federations don't allow them so you want to make sure you get used to doing it without.

Some people also like to use smelling salts to get themselves riled up before a lift. This activates the fight or flight response which can get your adrenaline pumping. However, if you're a calmer lifter than this might not help you much. You also need to be careful about the tubs exploding or leaking, they can cause very nasty burns.

The deadlift is often a feared movement due to people being concerned about their back. However,

good form and focused strength work will help protect against back injuries in the future and also help with posture and movement later on in life.
The deadlift uses the hamstrings, glutes, lower back, quadriceps, trapezius, lats, biceps, and forearms in order for you to complete it. The focus on these muscles differs depending on whether you do sumo or conventional.

One of the most controversial points amongst powerlifters is sumo vs conventional deadlifts. Conventional is the more common to the recreation gym goer. Just so you know what the difference is, here is a quick guide to the setups for each variation.

Conventional

- Start with your feet between hip and shoulder width.
- Have the bar over your bottom shoelace.
- Squat down to the bar with a flat back and grab the bar. (It is okay if your knees go ahead of the bar at this point).
- Your grip should be just outside of your feet.
- Pull yourself into the bar as you set your hips into position (this can take some messing around to find the perfect position).
- Push your legs into the floor as you pull the bar up and push your hips forward.

Sumo

- Your feet will be wide, very wide. So that when you do squat down your shins should be vertical, meaning your knees and ankles should be in alignment.
- Your toes should be pointed out at a diagonal angle.
- Your hand width is in line with your shoulders, so pretty much straight down.
- Your hip position is often the hard part to get right. You want them in a similar position to a conventional deadlift.
- You then, dig your heels into the floor as you pull (but do not yank) the bar off of the floor. It is likely to be slow off of the ground but it will move.
- As the bar passes your knees, lock them and then bring the hips forward, as you would in a conventional style also.

Variations

You will find many variations for each of these lifts. Such as...

- High bar and low bar squats.
- Front squats.
- Split Squats.
- Incline Bench Press.

- Dumbbell Bench Press.
- Reverse Grip Bench Press.
- Romanian Deadlifts.
- Stiff Legged Deadlifts.
- Etc.

All of these exercises will have their place within a good powerlifting training program, however, they are assistance exercises and are not necessarily what you will use on the platform. For this reason, the descriptions above have been for the competition specific movements.

Conclusion

This book was written with those in mind who want to give powerlifting a chance, but are unsure of what exactly it is. For those who have never quite tried their hand at out and out strength training but have rather stuck to the cardio section of the gym or have focused more upon isolation work or aesthetic and bodybuilding style of work.

By explaining the mindset involved in powerlifting, in both training and competing, while also defining and expanding upon what each lift is, we hope to have enlightened any complete beginners to trying a powerlifting program or maybe even a competition. If this book helps to get one person onto a platform anywhere in the world then we will have achieved our goal.

We hope that this provided a solid foundation for your first foray into the powerlifting world and that the basics of it are now clear to you. We also hope that you enjoyed reading and learning from this.

Thank You From Story Ninjas

Story Ninjas Publishing would like to thank you for reading our scary story anthology. We hope you found value in our book and would love to hear your feedback. Please provide your constructive criticism in a review on Amazon. Also feel free to share this book with your friends through various social media platforms.

Other Books by Story Ninjas

Story Ninjas Publishing hopes you enjoyed this short story anthology. You can find more of our products, by checking out our Amazon page.

About Story Ninjas

Story Ninjas Publishing is an independent book publisher. Our stories range from science fiction to paranormal romance. Our goal is to create stories that are not only entertaining but endearing. We believe engaging narrative can lead to personal growth. Through unforgettable characters and a powerful plot, we portray themes that are relevant to today's issues. Our hope is that readers find lessons they can apply to their everyday lives so that the stories live on through the actions of each person they touch. Additionally, we provide creative non-fiction books that are meant to serve as tools to help people solve everyday problems. We hope you find our products entertaining and helpful.

You can find Story Ninja's books on Kindle.

Follow Story Ninjas!!!
Website: www.Story-Ninjas.com
Email: Story-Ninjas@Story-Ninjas.com
Instagram: @StoryNinjas
Facebook: StoryNinjasHQ
LinkedIn: Story-Ninjas
Blogger: Story-NinjasHQ
Twitter: @StoryNinjas
Youtube: @StoryNinjas

Amazon: Story Ninjas
Podcast: Polymathics